# Graceful Ailments

## A Mindful Guide to Chronic Illness

# Table of Contents


1. Introduction . . . . . . . . . . . . . . . . . . . . . . . . . . . . . . . . . . . . . . . . . . . . 1

2. Understanding Chronic Illness: Definitions and Types . . . . . . . . . . 2

   2.1. The Broad Scope of Chronic Illness . . . . . . . . . . . . . . . . . . . . . . 2

   2.2. Living with Chronic Illness . . . . . . . . . . . . . . . . . . . . . . . . . . . 3

   2.3. The Battle of Acute vs Chronic Illness . . . . . . . . . . . . . . . . . . . 3

   2.4. Addressing the Invisible: Not All Chronic Illnesses are
Visible . . . . . . . . . . . . . . . . . . . . . . . . . . . . . . . . . . . . . . . . . . . . . 4

   2.5. Approach to Treatment and Management . . . . . . . . . . . . . . . . 4

3. One Size Does not Fit All: Personalizing Your Journey . . . . . . . . . . 6

   3.1. Your Journey, Your Narrative . . . . . . . . . . . . . . . . . . . . . . . . . 6

   3.2. Understanding the Role of Genetics . . . . . . . . . . . . . . . . . . . . 7

   3.3. Personalized Nutrition and Lifestyle . . . . . . . . . . . . . . . . . . . 7

   3.4. The Emotional Landscape and Chronic Illness . . . . . . . . . . . 8

   3.5. Shared Decision-making . . . . . . . . . . . . . . . . . . . . . . . . . . . . 8

4. The Art of Mindfulness: Cultivating Presence in Pain . . . . . . . . . . 10

   4.1. Understanding Mindfulness . . . . . . . . . . . . . . . . . . . . . . . . . 10

   4.2. Mindfulness and Chronic Illness: An Intersection . . . . . . . . 11

   4.3. The Building Blocks of Mindful Practice . . . . . . . . . . . . . . . . 11

   4.4. Incorporating Mindfulness in Daily Life . . . . . . . . . . . . . . . . 12

   4.5. Scaling the Peaks: Overcoming Mindfulness Challenges . . . . 13

   4.6. The Enriching Impact of Mindfulness . . . . . . . . . . . . . . . . . 13

5. Building Resilience: From Crisis to Possibility . . . . . . . . . . . . . . . . 15

   5.1. Resilience: Understanding the Concept . . . . . . . . . . . . . . . . . 15

   5.2. Cultivating Resilience: Break it down to Build it up . . . . . . . 16

   5.3. Getting to know your Resilience: The Inner Work . . . . . . . . . 16

   5.4. Leveraging external resources: The Reach Out . . . . . . . . . . . 16

   5.5. Resilience in the everyday: From Big Shifts to Micro
Practices . . . . . . . . . . . . . . . . . . . . . . . . . . . . . . . . . . . . . . . . . . . 17

5.6. Resilience: A Continuing Journey ....... 17

6. Whole Health Approach: Merging Conventional and Alternative Therapy ....... 19

6.1. Conventional Medicine: The Original Pillar ....... 19

6.2. Advancements in Conventional Medicine ....... 19

6.3. Alternative Therapies: The Budding Bloom ....... 20

6.4. The Salient Features of Alternative Therapies ....... 21

6.5. Integrating the Best of Both Worlds ....... 21

6.6. Benefits of an Integrated Approach ....... 22

6.7. In Conclusion ....... 22

7. Stigma and Social Reality: Navigating Life Beyond Treatment ... 24

7.1. The Nature of Stigma ....... 24

7.2. Counteracting Stigma and Building Resilience ....... 25

7.3. Fostering Communication: Conversations that Bridgel the Gap ....... 25

7.4. A World Beyond Labels: Embracing Your Identity ....... 26

7.5. Reframing Pains into Gains: Finding Silver Linings ....... 26

8. Tales Worth Telling: Inspiring Stories of Hope and Triumph ....... 28

8.1. The Rebirth: Cassandra's Journey ....... 28

8.2. True Grit: Jack's Undying Determination ....... 29

8.3. A Symphony in Silence: Laura's Dance with Deafness ....... 29

8.4. The Unseen Convoy: Johnathan's Invisible Illness ....... 30

8.5. New Purpose: From Wernicke's Aphasia to Art ....... 30

9. Family, Friends, and Partners: Thriving Relationships amidst Chronic Illness ....... 32

9.1. Navigating Family Dynamics ....... 32

9.2. Fostering Resilient Friendships ....... 33

9.3. Strengthening Partnership Bonds ....... 33

9.4. The Gift Of Empathy ....... 34

9.5. Transforming Relationships ....... 34

10. Finances and Future: A Practical Guide to Managing Long-term Care . . . . . . . . . . . . . . . . . . . . . . . . . . . . . . . . . . . . . . . . . 36

    10.1. Budgeting Basics . . . . . . . . . . . . . . . . . . . . . . . . . . . . . . 36

    10.2. Insurance Insights . . . . . . . . . . . . . . . . . . . . . . . . . . . . 37

    10.3. Potential Financial Assistance . . . . . . . . . . . . . . . . . . 38

    10.4. Planning for the Future . . . . . . . . . . . . . . . . . . . . . . . 38

    10.5. Legal Considerations . . . . . . . . . . . . . . . . . . . . . . . . . 38

11. Living Passionately: Finding Purpose and Fulfillment in Chronic Illness . . . . . . . . . . . . . . . . . . . . . . . . . . . . . . . . . . . . . 40

    11.1. The Pursuit of Purpose . . . . . . . . . . . . . . . . . . . . . . . 40

    11.2. Embracing Fulfillment . . . . . . . . . . . . . . . . . . . . . . . . 41

    11.3. The Power of Connection . . . . . . . . . . . . . . . . . . . . . . 41

    11.4. Defying Defeat: Exhibiting Resilience . . . . . . . . . . . . 42

    11.5. Cultivating Mindfulness . . . . . . . . . . . . . . . . . . . . . . . 42

    11.6. The Road Less Traveled . . . . . . . . . . . . . . . . . . . . . . . 43

# Chapter 1. Introduction

Welcome to Graceful Ailments: A Mindful Guide to Chronic Illness. This Special Report explores the uncharted territory of finding calm, peace, and resilience amidst the whirlwind of chronic disease. Crafted with care, empathy, and in-depth research, it is designed to spark hope for those navigating this complex terrain. Our narrative transcends medical jargon, converging medical insights with the lived experiences of real people. It is an unexpectedly heartening and uplifting journey, one that unearths the transformative potential of living mindfully with chronic illness. Don't just survive your circumstances - buy this guide to uncover wisdom, resilience and a renewed zest for life against all odds.

# Chapter 2. Understanding Chronic Illness: Definitions and Types

Chronic illnesses are diseases or conditions that persist for more than three months, often lasting a person's lifetime. However, the definition of chronic illness is far more intricate when we consider the multifaceted effects it can have on an individual's life.

The Centers for Disease Control and Prevention (CDC), the leading national public health institute of the United States, reveals that six in ten adults in the US have a chronic disease, while four in ten adults have two or more. These statistics are staggering, given the long-term persisting nature of these illnesses, which tend to leave individuals grappling with symptoms and side-effects that extend beyond the physical and medical field.

## 2.1. The Broad Scope of Chronic Illness

There are countless types of chronic illnesses, each unique in its presentation, symptoms, and the treatment required. They are commonly grouped into the following categories:

1. Cardiovascular diseases (such as heart disease and stroke)

2. Cancers

3. Chronic respiratory diseases (such as COPD and asthma)

4. Diabetes

5. Mental health conditions (such as depression, anxiety, and bipolar disorder)

6. Auto-immune diseases (such as lupus, multiple sclerosis, and rheumatoid arthritis)

7. Neurodegenerative disorders (such as Parkinson's disease and Alzheimer's)

8. Chronic pain conditions (such as fibromyalgia and chronic fatigue syndrome)

9. Digestive disorders (such as irritable bowel syndrome and Crohn's disease)

Some are more common than others, while some are rare or lesser-known - often presenting challenges in diagnosis, treatment, and management.

## 2.2. Living with Chronic Illness

Living with chronic illness often involves intricately managing symptoms, health regimens, medications, and lifestyle changes. This management is rarely straightforward - one day a person may feel relatively well, and the next, they may be incapacitated by symptoms. This fluctuation is one of the defining features of chronic illness.

It has profound effects on all aspects of life, often leading to changes in work ability, social relationships, hobbies, and even basic daily tasks. The toll on mental health can also be significant, with many people experiencing anxiety, depression, or other mental health conditions in conjunction with their physical symptoms.

## 2.3. The Battle of Acute vs Chronic Illness

Whist acute illnesses such as the flu or a cold have a clear beginning and end, chronic illnesses persist. It is essential to distinguish between the two because treatment and coping strategies differ significantly. In acute conditions, the primary goal is usually recovery, while in chronic illnesses, the focus often shifts to managing symptoms and maintaining the highest possible quality of life, given the persistent nature of the condition.

## 2.4. Addressing the Invisible: Not All Chronic Illnesses are Visible

Recognizing that not all chronic illnesses are visible is vital. Many can significantly affect a person's daily life and functioning while leaving few, if any, outward signs. Conditions like chronic pain, mental illness, and fibromyalgia can be largely 'invisible', leading to misunderstandings, stigma, and a lack of support. People dealing with invisible conditions often experience the added struggle of having to 'prove' their illness to others, placing an additional burden on their shoulders.

## 2.5. Approach to Treatment and Management

Treating and managing chronic illness is often complex, requiring a multifaceted approach. This approach may include various treatments, such as medications, surgeries, therapies, lifestyle changes, and a wealth of self-care strategies.

Evidence from the field of Mind-Body medicine suggests that mind-body practices can significantly benefit people living with chronic illness. Techniques such as mindfulness meditation, yoga, tai chi, and cognitive behavioral therapy can help manage symptoms, improve mental health, improve quality of life, and even influence the course of illness.

This report aims to take you, the reader, through the journey of understanding chronic illness, its spectrum, and exploring these alternative mind-body avenues that have shown promising results, focusing not just on the challenge posed by chronic illness but also on the hope and resilience that can be found amidst the struggle.

# Chapter 3. One Size Does not Fit All: Personalizing Your Journey

Navigating the intricate maze of chronic illness is a deeply personal journey. Unlike an acute ailment that typically has a prescribed roadmap towards recovery, chronic conditions engender a wide spectrum of experiences. Each person's body reacts differently to the illness and treatment, making the path to symptom management and wellbeing unique for every individual.

## 3.1. Your Journey, Your Narrative

Within the medical community, there is a growing recognition that each person's narrative lies at the heart of their treatment. The illness is not a detached entity, but an intricate part of the person. Knowing the story of their disease—the unique symptomology, the distinct impact on daily life, the specific stressors—can provide valuable insights for healthcare providers in tailoring appropriate treatment plans.

Creating your narrative is an essential first step towards personalized healthcare. Start by noting down symptom patterns, emotional responses, triggers, reliefs, and coping mechanisms. But remember, your narrative isn't limited to your illness alone. It should also include your emotional well-being, personal life, relationships, work situation, and any other aspects that play a significant role in your overall health.

## 3.2. Understanding the Role of Genetics

Our genetic make-up can significantly influence the way chronic diseases manifest and how our bodies respond to treatments. Researchers are exploring the realm of "personalized medicine", where your genetic profile can help doctors predict the efficacy of certain drugs or treatments. Genetic tests today can provide insights into potential medication side-effects, dosage requirements, and even prognostic outcomes.

While this field holds great promise, it's also important to understand its limitations. Genetics is just one piece of the puzzle. Environmental factors, lifestyle habits, co-existing health conditions, and even the state of our gut flora can play significant roles in disease progression and responsiveness to treatment.

## 3.3. Personalized Nutrition and Lifestyle

The adage "Let food be thy medicine" becomes particularly relevant when dealing with chronic illnesses. Nutrition plays a central role in chronic disease management, influencing both the manifestation of symptoms and the body's ability to cope with them. Often, people dealing with chronic disease find that certain foods can trigger or exacerbate symptoms, while others can provide unexpected relief.

Opt for a personalized nutrition plan instead of following generic diet plans. Seek the help of a professional dietitian or nutritionist who acknowledges the complexity of your condition and tailors a nutrition plan that caters to your specific needs and challenges.

Keep in mind, what we consume is just as important as how we live. Sleep, physical activity, and stress management—these lifestyle factors have a profound impact on your health outcomes. Work with healthcare professionals to help customize a lifestyle plan that aligns with your medical needs and personal circumstances.

## 3.4. The Emotional Landscape and Chronic Illness

The impact of chronic illness reaches far beyond physical symptoms. It permeates into our emotional spaces, affecting well-being, mental health, and our relationships. Therefore, a realistic treatment plan cannot ignore emotional health.

Engaging with a psychologist or mental health professional can help navigate the emotional labyrinth of chronic illness. Therapy can equip you with psychological tools and coping mechanisms that support resilience and enhance quality of life.

Emotional care becomes an act of self-affirmation, acknowledging that you are more than your illness. By weaving emotional care into your personalized journey, you create a narrative that supports physical healing while concurrently promoting emotional well-being.

## 3.5. Shared Decision-making

Personalized care thrives on shared decision-making, a process where you and your healthcare providers collaborate to make healthcare decisions that align with your preferences and values. This involves documenting treatment goals, discussing potential benefits and drawbacks, and considering alternatives.

Remember, shared decision-making is not about being a passive recipient of medical information, but a collaborator in your healthcare journey. This equitable partnership fosters personalized care, as it recognizes and respects your individuality and experience, leading to better health outcomes.

Embarking on a journey with chronic illness may seem daunting, confusing, and isolating. Always remember, there isn't a one-size-fits-all solution for chronic illness. Your journey is uniquely yours. By bringing personalized care into your treatment, you honor your individuality and tap into your inner strength, enabling you to flourish, even in adversity.

# Chapter 4. The Art of Mindfulness: Cultivating Presence in Pain

Let's embark upon a journey — a journey where we unravel the essence of mindful living. The journey might seem daunting given our circumstances, but it invites us to tap into an untapped reservoir: the art of being present, even in the midst of pain.

## 4.1. Understanding Mindfulness

Mindfulness, at its core, signifies an overarching awareness of our present experience, a deep-rooted acceptance of the shell we embody, and the world around us —yes, even the pain we incessantly endure. Derived from centuries-old Buddhist meditation practices, it beckons us to exist in the moment, observe our thoughts and sensations nonjudgmentally, and inspire a crucial shift in our perspective towards reality.

However, mindfulness is not about dismissing or defying the pain. It's about acknowledging it, co-existing with it, and utilizing it as a tool for unprecedented understanding and empathy. It invites us to the rarely explored realm of quiet strength, resilience, and hope, enveloped by an aura of peace that pain inevitably tries to veil.

# 4.2. Mindfulness and Chronic Illness: An Intersection

Chronic illness often forces us into a state of dread and despair. We repeatedly find ourselves trapped in the gloomy backroads of our minds—constantly ruminating, contemplating the irreversibility of our circumstances. These moments call for mindfulness, to propel us out of the darkened alleys and into the sunshine of acceptance and tranquility.

Crucially, mindfulness may not transform our condition, yet it has the potential to evolve our reactions towards it. Studies reflect its positive outcomes on chronic pain, anxiety, depression, and life satisfaction, as it brings into light the often forgotten ingredients of living—a sense of purpose, a tad of joy, or simply, long-lasting calmness.

# 4.3. The Building Blocks of Mindful Practice

Embarking upon the journey of mindfulness may seem labyrinthine, yet it starts with an incredibly simple step — paying attention.

- Awareness: Start by acknowledging the labyrinth of emotions — fear, anger, despair — coiling around your chronic illness. It's about noticing these sentiments and comprehending their fleeting nature.

- Non-Judgment: More than observing, mindfulness insists on non-judgmental observation. Do not label your thoughts as 'good' or 'bad'. Detach your self-worth from your circumstances.

- Acceptance: Acceptance doesn't mean surrender; it means

understanding that pain is a part of your narrative, not your entire story. It's about cultivating self-empathy, creating space between yourself and your suffering.

- Presence: Strive for ongoing presence, continually tether your attentiveness to the here-and-now. Abstain from anticipating pain or dwelling on past suffering.

# 4.4. Incorporating Mindfulness in Daily Life

Mindfulness is not limited to meditation—it seeps into every facet of existence.

- Mindful Breathing: Reconnect with your breath. Inhale calmly, exhale gently. It is a constant, soothing reminder that you are alive and present.

- Mindful Eating: Cherish each nibble, each gulp. Relish the myriad textures, flavors, the sheer joy of nourishing your body.

- Mindful Activities: Find solace in daily routines. The rhythmic wash of dishes, the gentle flip of a book page, or the warm cascade of shower water—fleeting moments of everyday serenity.

- Mindful Conversations: Listen patiently, respond empathetically. Make meaningful connections, nurture relationships — it's therapeutic.

# 4.5. Scaling the Peaks: Overcoming Mindfulness Challenges

As we embark upon our mindfulness journey, we might encounter hurdles. Here are a few ways to deal with them:

- Set achievable goals: Don't chase instantaneous enlightenment. Start small, appreciate your little victories, and gradually deepen your mindfulness practice.

- Be patient: Mindfulness is not a quick fix, it's a step-by-step process. Remember, healing is seldom linear, and so is mindfulness.

- Seek support: Mindfulness, though a personal journey, doesn't have to be undertaken alone. Consider joining a mindfulness-based support group or seeking guidance from a mindfulness instructor.

# 4.6. The Enriching Impact of Mindfulness

Mindfulness, when woven into the threadwork of our lives, triggers an awakening — an understanding that chronic illness does not solely define us. It helps us rise above our circumstances and comprehend that amid the vortex of perpetual pain, we can find fragments of joy, sparks of resilience, and glimmers of hope. It might not eradicate our pain, but it certainly illuminates the darkened alleyways, presenting us with an entirely new perspective — a mindful landscape that fosters growth not despite, but because of, our pain.

Now, you are equipped with the necessary knowledge — breathe, observe, accept, and be in the present. Navigate the waters of your life with renewed vigor and grace. The path might be uncharted, and the waters might be rough, but within you reserves a strength undefined and a spirit unconquered. A mindfulness journey with chronic pain is undeniably challenging, but simultaneously, it's an unexpected odyssey of self-discovery, acceptance, and serenity. Experience your world not through the prism of chronic illness, but through the lens of mindfulness.

# Chapter 5. Building Resilience: From Crisis to Possibility

A life-altering illness invariably sets in motion a chaotic tumble of emotions, a myriad of chaotic feelings laced with fear, uncertainty, and confusion. These initial naturally reactive emotions can envelop and consume a person, rendering them incapable of seeing through the opacity to the potential for growth encapsulated within. Resilience, a key quality in navigating the challenges accompanying chronic illness, starts to truly blossom when one reframes the crisis as a passage to possibility.

## 5.1. Resilience: Understanding the Concept

Resilience is a term waving high in the flag of psychological discourse. From overcoming personal trauma to navigating life-altering incidents such as chronic illness, resilience stands as a crucial determinant of how effectively one adapts and thrives.

Undeniably, the experience of being diagnosed with a chronic illness can trigger a psychological crisis. Within this space, resilience is often the buoy that helps keep an individual from sinking in the dark waters of despair and fear. But, what do we mean when we say 'resilience'?

Resilience is not about being impervious to life's hardships. Rather, it represents the ability to 'bounce back' from adversities, the capacity to adapt and move forward despite setbacks. It involves drawing on inner strengths, harnessing supporting resources, and nurturing a future-forward perspective to navigate the challenges effectively.

## 5.2. Cultivating Resilience: Break it down to Build it up

The cultivation of resilience is by no means a trivial task. While the process serves a different purpose for everyone, there are certain universal aspects that work towards building resilience.

## 5.3. Getting to know your Resilience: The Inner Work

*Lastly, foster the practice of self-care. This encompasses physical care, managing symptoms with respected medical advice but also mental, emotional and spiritual self-nourishment.*

Beyond universal strategies for building resilience, each journey is personal and unique. At its heart, resilience is deeply tied to personal practices and perspectives - what meditative or therapeutic routines work for you? Resilience building is a lifelong commitment to inner work, to fostering a relationship with oneself that is grounded in authenticity and patience.

## 5.4. Leveraging external resources: The Reach Out

*By developing your spiritual intelligence: Cultivating a connection to something larger than oneself, regardless of religious affiliations, can provide a profound sense of meaning and direction especially during challenging times.*

A critical but often overlooked component of building resilience is leveraging external resources. Indeed, resilience rises from the intertwining vines of inner strength and external support.

# 5.5. Resilience in the everyday: From Big Shifts to Micro Practices

*Seek professional advice: Access the guidance of pertinent professionals, be they doctors, dietitians, therapists, or social workers. These external resources can provide practical coping techniques and tools for your resilience toolkit.*

Resilience isn't merely a grand, sweeping shift in consciousness. It's a journey made up of tiny steps, everyday practices, and small pivots in perspective. The art of acknowledging and appreciating small triumphs, for instance, noticing the strength you demonstrated in managing a symptom flare-up can help build resilience.

Similarly, tools like mindfulness and meditation, gentle movement or yoga, journaling or art, can serve as practical paths to resilience, fostering a sense of calm and stability amidst the storm of chronic illness. Small, manageable changes in your daily routine can become the soil from which your resilience begins to grow.

# 5.6. Resilience: A Continuing Journey

Living with chronic illness presents an ongoing test of resilience. There are no shortcuts, miraculous cures, or overnight transformations. Instead, resilience arises from perseverance, determination, patience, and most importantly, a deep-seated commitment to oneself.

Whether chronic illness has been a longstanding chapter or a recent entry in your life story, remember the power of resilience rests within you. Transfigure the crisis into a passage of discovery and growth. Resilience is not merely about surviving but thriving in your journey, embracing possibility amidst adversity, and continuing to find, renew and celebrate your ardor for life. In the earnest endeavor of building resilience and transmuting pain into power, you are your greatest ally.

# Chapter 6. Whole Health Approach: Merging Conventional and Alternative Therapy

Is it not with a sense of bewilderment that we often approach the idea of illness? However, it is time to go beyond the traditional framework and explore a wholesome view of health that embraces both conventional and alternative therapies. This integrative approach builds on the mutual strengths of these two worlds to bring about the best possible health outcomes.

## 6.1. Conventional Medicine: The Original Pillar

A solid foundation in any healthcare approach is the tried and tested realm of conventional medicine. This mode of treatment, largely attributed to Western science, focuses on the manifestation of diseases within the body and its curative aspects.

It places primary emphasis on the physical symptoms of the disease rather than looking at the issue from a holistic standpoint. With its objective, evidence-based approach, it has led to many crucial breakthroughs in healthcare, including successful treatment plans for numerous diseases.

## 6.2. Advancements in Conventional Medicine

Over the years, conventional medicine is seen to have advanced impressively. Biomedical technologies and pharmacological solutions have immensely contributed to the evolution of treatment protocols. The use of ultrasounds, CT scans, genetic testing, personalized medication plans, and more, offers a high degree of precision in disease detection and management.

In conjunction with this progress, the development of a wide gamut of pharmaceuticals has been paralleled, adding up to the arsenal against illness. Ranging from vaccines to chemotherapies, drug therapies have substantially increased medical robustness.

Traditional medicine rightfully holds a pillar position in our health system. However, it does also possess limitations. Conventional methods often focus on symptom alleviation, sometimes neglecting the overall well-being of patients and failing to address the causative stressors impacting health.

# 6.3. Alternative Therapies: The Budding Bloom

Alternative therapies, often considered the 'other' in the world of medicine, refers to diverse health practices, products, and systems that are typically not part of institutionalized medical training. The landscape is abundant with treatments such as herbal medicine, acupuncture, yoga, meditation, and diet control, among others.

This approach is gaining favor due to its focus on rebalancing the energy flow in the body and promoting a strong mind-body connection. It encourages an individual to be conscientious of their lifestyle and habits, fostering an active role in their own health management.

# 6.4. The Salient Features of Alternative Therapies

The basis of most alternative therapies lies in ancient philosophies and traditional practices. They tend to take a person-centered approach, treat every individual as a unique being, and view health as a state of balance among body, mind, and spirit.

Some alternative therapies, like Traditional Chinese Medicine (TCM) and Ayurveda, operate on concepts like the flow of vital energy (Qi in TCM, Prana in Ayurveda) and balance of elemental constituents (Yin-Yang in TCM, Doshas in Ayurveda). Others, like yoga and meditation, emphasize mental tranquility and focus.

However, quantifying the benefits of alternative therapies has been a challenge due to the lack of comprehensive, controlled studies and the relative subjectivity of results. Despite this, a growing number of patients are turning to alternative medicine for chronic conditions, particularly where conventional methods have not yielded desired results.

# 6.5. Integrating the Best of Both Worlds

While both modes of healing hold their own significant advantages, a combined approach could revolutionize medicine as we know it today. A whole health approach would merge both these worlds, integrating conventional diagnostics and treatments with alternative therapies to create a more rounded, comprehensive healthcare plan.

# 6.6. Benefits of an Integrated Approach

This integrative approach offers numerous benefits. For starters, it allows for individualized care plans tailored to each patient's unique needs and circumstances. It considers the totality of the person - their physical symptoms, emotional state, lifestyle, and spiritual beliefs - to address the root cause of the disease.

Moreover, an active involvement of the patient is promoted in such an approach, fostering a sense of control and responsibility over their own health. Effective communication between healthcare providers and patients illuminates the path of this journey, bridging the gaps that could exist in understanding the disease and its treatment.

Finally, through its complementary nature, this approach might help mitigate the side effects of conventional treatments. For instance, yoga or acupuncture could alleviate the nausea associated with chemotherapy, or meditation could aid in managing the chronic pain of arthritis.

# 6.7. In Conclusion

The incorporation of complementary and alternative practices with conventional medicine signifies a substantive shift in healthcare culture. As research continues to illuminate the benefits of a holistic health approach, it becomes our responsibility as healthcare providers, patients, and advocates, to nurture this integrated model and bring it into reach of those who need it most.

Remember, managing chronic illness is not just about treating symptoms. It is about acknowledging the interconnectedness of our bodies and minds, understanding the intrinsic ability to heal, and cultivating a deep sense of well-being even amidst these challenges.

This comprehensive mind-body approach does not merely aspire to healing, but to well-being, resilience, and universally accessible health care for all.

23

# Chapter 7. Stigma and Social Reality: Navigating Life Beyond Treatment

A diagnosis of chronic illness ushers in a bewildering array of medical realities. Painful treatments, expensive medications, lifestyle adjustments, and countless consultations become the new normal. However, we seldom discuss a ubiquitous and yet elusive challenge chronic disease warriors confront: the stigma.

Social stigma, simply put, refers to the disapproval, rejection, or discrimination by others based on a particular attribute, in this case, being diagnosed with a chronic illness. Understanding and addressing stigma is vital as it shapes our experiences in profound ways, often exacerbating the physical symptoms and emotional duress of a chronic ailment.

## 7.1. The Nature of Stigma

Stigma severs connections, creates solitude, and drives individual into the shadows. It happens when society imparts derogatory attributes on individuals with a chronic illness, causing them to feel diminished or spoiled in some way. Social interactions become stifled, leading to a sense of isolation and alienation even in familiar environments. The disturbing reality is that stigma often comes from loved ones, colleagues, or people who should ideally provide support and reassurance.

## 7.2. Counteracting Stigma and Building Resilience

Fighting stigma requires resilience. Resilience, or the ability to bounce back from adversity, can be nurtured. Here lies the uncelebrated beauty of life with a chronic illness: it empowers you to develop resilience, like a muscle, through daily battles against the disease itself and the stigma that shrouds it.

Discover your internal locus of control, which is the belief that you can influence events and outcomes in your life. It's a mindset shift from being a 'patient' to becoming an active participant in your journey to wellness. Cultivating this sense of personal agency demystifies disease and gives you a sense of command over your circumstances.

## 7.3. Fostering Communication: Conversations that Bridgel the Gap

In mitigating stigma, communication plays a pivotal role. Acknowledge your feelings and share them with a trusted confidant. Transparency fosters understanding, and reaching out can help you forge real connections instead of feeling alienated. Engage in conversations about your conditions, symptoms, fears, and discomfort.

Volunteering for a local support group or engaging online in relevant forums can also offer a sense of community. You are not alone in your struggles, and joining such communities facilitates sharing experiences, knowledge, coping strategies. It provides an environment replete with empathy and understanding, constituting a healing vista in itself.

## 7.4. A World Beyond Labels: Embracing Your Identity

It's important to remember that you're not defined by your disease. By focusing on your channels of resilience and mastering your locus of control, you can see past the illness and reestablish your identity beyond the labels of disease. This is not to undermine the disease's impact, but to refuse to let it eclipse your identity.

Chronic illness inevitably becomes a part of your life narrative, but it's just a chapter, not the entire book. Identify your strengths, passions, and skills and integrate them into your identity. Your illness is a part of you, not your entirety. By grounding yourself in an identity larger than your illness, you can redefine the narrative.

## 7.5. Reframing Pains into Gains: Finding Silver Linings

The concept of 'reframing' is a potent psychological tool that has been instrumental in helping numerous people navigate their chronic illness journey. Reframing essentially means consciously choosing to interpret a situation or experience in a constructive or positive way.

Chronic illness may bring pain, but it can also induce personal growth, self-knowledge, empathy, and perspective shifts. Each journey with chronic disease is uniquely transformative and transformative experiences, for all their adversity, are beautiful. Cherish the silver linings when they appear, and seek them when they hide.

Ending the chapter here, we understand that not every day will be easy, and neither will every interaction. But through resilience and mindful living, stigma can be faced, and hopefully, eradicated. Chronic illness may change you, but remember – change is not always a lesser. Change can mean growth, wisdom, and an expanded perspective on life. On days when stigma weighs you down, remember your innate resilience and your ability to rise, time and again.

# Chapter 8. Tales Worth Telling: Inspiring Stories of Hope and Triumph

Our initial steps towards understanding the essence of living with chronic illness bring us to remarkable tales - unique life-stories constructed within the churning vortex of chronic health issues. These stories form the canvas on which we can perceive the struggle, resilience, hope, and the triumph of the human spirit.

## 8.1. The Rebirth: Cassandra's Journey

Cassandra was an active sportswoman, her days filled with rigorous training and joyful exertion. However, her vibrant life rhythm began to ebb away when she was diagnosed with rheumatoid arthritis at the tender age of 22.

Tasked with the challenge of adapting to the new reality, Cassandra underwent a metamorphosis. She practiced mindfulness meditation, focusing her attention on her body without judgment, and, importantly, without resistance to her new symptom experiences. Through this process, she discovered a newfound appreciation for yoga and tai chi, both of which contributed to her fitness and mental stamina.

Rising from her ashes, Cassandra is now a certified yoga instructor. She sees her diagnosis not as a failure, but as a pivot towards accessing a deeper part of her being that she might never have accessed: a transformative shift through her ailment.

# 8.2. True Grit: Jack's Undying Determination

In the tapestry of chronic illness narratives, Jack's story stands out. Struggling from his teenage years with type 1 diabetes, the disease often posed hurdles in his endeavors.

Doctors had warned of the dangers that his love for mountain climbing posed. However, Jack, with staunch determination, altered his approach to managing his illness. He meticulously tracked his insulin levels, planned his diet, and worked out with determination harder than ever before. Climbing mountains was no more a dream but a reality he lived.

Despite the countless blackouts and the relentless fight to balance his insulin on his climbs, Jack is now legendary within the climbing community and beyond. His endeavors echo that it's not the severity of illness, but the intensity of grit that defines us.

# 8.3. A Symphony in Silence: Laura's Dance with Deafness

Laura was a sophomore at Juilliard when sudden sensorineural hearing loss struck her. Crushing her dreams of becoming a professional violinist, Laura's life seemed to lose its harmony.

However, Laura didn't let the disheartening event bog her down. She began exploring dance - a skill she had dabbled as a hobby. In tune with the rhythm, Laura found solace in the vibrations. She experienced the world of sound through the dimensions of movement.

Defying all odds, Laura became a ballerina and formed a dance company for deaf and hard-of-hearing dancers. Her tale is a beautiful dance of resilience, refracting the vulnerability and strength that lies deeply intertwined within the human spirit facing adversity.

## 8.4. The Unseen Convoy: Johnathan's Invisible Illness

Johnathan, living with Crohn's disease, found himself enduring an ailment that the world couldn't see, but he felt with an intensity that was hard to ignore.

Stigma coupled with the debilitating physical torment of this invisible illness pushed him towards self-isolation. It was then, in the mire of his agony, Johnathan found solace in writing.

Expressing his experiences with his unperceived symptoms, he found an external means to shape his ordeal. And as a beacon of hope, he crafted a blog, sharing his story, his struggles, his triumphs over his condition.

Johnathan's blog became a sanctuary, a space of understanding for many traversing a similar path. His story instills the belief that even within suffering, there exists the capacity to uplift, inspire and connect.

## 8.5. New Purpose: From Wernicke's Aphasia to Art

As a renowned barrister, David had a command of language to which many aspire. However, following a severe stroke, he was diagnosed with Wernicke's aphasia, significantly impairing his speech.

Dejected by the loss of his oratory abilities, David was drawn towards art therapy. He discovered a unique peace in the fusion of colors, the strokes that represented his vision so intimately and purely.

David turned his world around, exhibiting his artwork which spoke volumes, standing testament to his renewed passion and cherished resilience. His transformation communicates the power of alternative expression and the compelling journey of reinvention amid adversity.

These stories, though scarred with chronic ailments, bear witness to the extraordinary adaptive capabilities and resilience of the human spirit. Embracing the trials of their physical conditions, each person has woven their adversity into a tapestry of triumph and transformation. Their tales are not just stories of struggle and survival, but powerful metaphors of hope and transcendence that illuminate the intricate and compelling path of living mindfully with chronic illness.

# Chapter 9. Family, Friends, and Partners: Thriving Relationships amidst Chronic Illness

Living with chronic disease can feel like navigating an intricate labyrinth. Still, it does not have to be a solitary journey. Our familial bonds, friendships, and relationships with our partners can be a beacon, offering support, understanding, and love, even amidst the storms of chronic illness. They can illuminate our path, turning hardship into resilience. However, consistent communication, empathy, and mutual respect are essential for maintaining these relationships.

## 9.1. Navigating Family Dynamics

Families form the nucleus of our social existence. Hence, witnessing a family member endure a chronic illness is inherently challenging. In addition to the emotional toll, it requires frequent modifications of familial roles and dynamics.

Open dialogue forms the cornerstone of mutual understanding within a family set-up. Start by explaining your illness, needs, and limitations. Keep them abreast of doctor visits, treatment plans, and progress. This transparency helps in minimizing misunderstandings, fostering collective resilience.

Yet, it's equally important to provide space for the emotional responses of the family. Encourage them to express their feelings, concerns, and fears. Remember, while your experience is unique, chronic illness affects everyone in the family on different levels.

A family that communicates well will also make adjustments as necessary. Flexibility can soften the blow of chronic illness on daily activities and routines.

# 9.2. Fostering Resilient Friendships

*include::common/list-learn-to-communicate.adoc[]*

Living with chronic illness may change the nature of friendships, often straining both old bonds and the ability to create new ones. Distancing may occur when friends don't immediately understand your limitations or struggle to grapple with your illness. Keep in mind that this is often due to ignorance rather than malice.

To maintain and foster resilient friendships:

- Be candid about your illness and its everyday impact

- Encourage them to ask questions to understand better

- Educate them about your condition, patiently and consistently

- Foster empathy by sharing your experiences and struggles, thus building stronger bonds

Despite your best efforts, friendships might still change, and some may inevitably fade. This is a harsh reality of chronic illness. Yet, such changes may also lead to discovering the core group of friends who stand unwavering in their support.

# 9.3. Strengthening Partnership Bonds

When a partner is diagnosed with a chronic disease, it invariably adds a new dimension to the relationship- an unforeseen challenge that both partners need to navigate. The coping mechanisms vary widely, with reactions including fear, anger, guilt, or even denial.

The following strategies can mitigate these challenges:

- Regular, open, and clear communication about the disease and its implications
- Joint appointments to doctor visits or therapy sessions
- Active involvement in care regimes
- Caring for the caregiver, acknowledging their stresses and emotional needs too

And most importantly, never allowing the disease to define the relationship.

# 9.4. The Gift Of Empathy

*include::common/list-caring-for-the-caregiver.adoc[]*

While chronic illness challenges relationships at every turn, it also presents a unique opportunity to cultivate empathy. Having a loved one grappling with a chronic disease nudges us towards greater understanding and compassion.

Both societal dialogues and educational initiatives can play catalytic roles in spreading empathetic awareness about chronic illnesses. Establishing supportive communities and encouraging wider societal engagement will also contribute to a more inclusive understanding.

# 9.5. Transforming Relationships

Chronic illness can indeed drastically transform relationships. However, remember that change isn't always negative. It often presents an opportunity for growth and increased resilience. It encourages the development of a deeper understanding, empathy, and mutual respect in relationships.

Even though living with chronic disease is a pathway sprinkled with sorrows and challenges, it also grants an idiosyncratic lens to view life—one where relationships can thrive amidst adversity. It's about finding the delicate balance between dependence and independence, expressing love and gratitude, embracing change, and savoring the moment. Through this tumultuous journey, remember, relationships aren't just about surviving, they're about thriving.

At the end of the day, chronic illness does not determine the love, care, and connections in life. We do.

# Chapter 10. Finances and Future: A Practical Guide to Managing Long-term Care

Living with a chronic illness isn't merely about managing one's health, but encompasses a host of practical aspects as well. One crucial element that can cause significant stress is the financial implications and future planning aspects of long-term care. It might often feel overwhelming, but carefully planned financial decisions can alleviate much of the strain.

## 10.1. Budgeting Basics

Understanding your living situation as a chronic illness patient is the starting point to financial planning. These include the requirements of your healthcare, your current monthly budget, and necessary adjustments to your lifestyle to accommodate the cost of long-term care. Evaluate your essential and nonessential expenses, then prioritize accordingly.

Understanding the cost of your illness helps to set a realistic budget, keeping in mind the variable nature of some medical expenses. Be sure to budget for medication, treatments, therapies, doctor's appointments, and transportation costs, among others. Also, consider potential loss of income due to medical leave or decrease in professional activity.

Lists and tables can be your best ally in this task. Construct a comprehensive list of your regular incomes, expenses, and healthcare costs. This measure can help you get a grip on where your money is going and plan accordingly.

```
|===
|Income Source|Amount|Frequency
|Job (primary)|$3000|Monthly
|Freelance Work|$500|Irregular
|Rent Income|$700|Monthly
|===
```

```
|===
|Regular Expenses|Amount|Frequency
|Rent/Mortgage|$1200|Monthly
|Grocery|$300|Weekly
|Utilities|$200|Monthly
|Car Payments|$300|Monthly
|===
```

```
|===
|Healthcare Expenses |Cost|Frequency
|Prescription Medication|$80|Bi-weekly
|Physiotherapy |$120|Weekly
|Doctor Appointments|$100|Monthly
|Travel to Appointments|$50|Weekly
|===
```

# 10.2. Insurance Insights

Insurance is a crucial pillar of your financial planning. Understand thoroughly the specifics of your health insurance policy. Be proactive in clarifying any ambiguous areas. Health insurance affects all your medical costs, so comprehending your policy's inclusions, exclusions, deductibles, and out-of-pocket maximums can help plan your budget more effectively.

Don't overlook long-term care insurance. This coverage can crucially help in situations like adult day-care, in-home care, or nursing home costs. Ensure you are clear on the specifics of what this insurance presents. Also, keep an eye open for any disability insurance you might have through your employer. These policies can help offset lost income in the event of decreased work ability.

## 10.3. Potential Financial Assistance

Depending on your specific circumstances, consider finding financial assistance. Various grants, programs, and nonprofit initiatives support chronic illness patients. Investigate all potential options - don't let pride get in the way of seeking help. There is no shame in needing support; it's a part of human life.

## 10.4. Planning for the Future

A part of managing your finances involves planning for the future. Consider factors such as retirement, children's education, vacation funds, or any significant future expenses. Working with a financial advisor who has experience with chronic illnesses can offer valuable insights. They may suggest, for example, some life insurance and annuity products which could provide guaranteed income.

## 10.5. Legal Considerations

When managing finances with a chronic illness, legal considerations often arise. Consider establishing a will, living will, and assigning a durable power of attorney. These legal documents protect your interests should your health interfere with your decision-making ability.

To conclude, while managing finances with chronic illness can feel overwhelming, it is possible to achieve strong financial health by planning well and seeking guidance. The key lies in understanding your unique situation and making informed, thoughtful decisions. Balancing your health and financial future might seem challenging initially, but with resilience and wisdom, you can navigate your journey with a calm and steady heart.

# Chapter 11. Living Passionately: Finding Purpose and Fulfillment in Chronic Illness

Living with chronic illness often feels like a journey without a map, an uncharted and treacherous landscape where every tentative step forward might herald either an unexpected pitfall or a springboard towards new insights and opportunities. But amid the many challenges and obstacles you may encounter, finding purpose and fulfillment is not only possible but can even contribute to your overall well-being.

## 11.1. The Pursuit of Purpose

Many of us find purpose through activities or roles that bring us joy and align with our values. As someone with a chronic illness, your paths to these may be different, but that doesn't mean they're less significant or fulfilling. Purpose isn't a destination, it's a process, and chronic illness doesn't end this journey, but it does transform it.

Take some time, quiet space, and gentle self-compassion to ask yourself: What roles and activities have I been passionate about in the past? What am I curious about now? What creates a flutter in my chest, a spark in my eye, or a peaceful sense of alignment with my deepest values? Write these down, reflect on them, talk with trusted friends, therapists, or mentors. Use this as a lighthouse to direct your future actions, adapting when necessary but always keeping the beam in sight.

Bill, a former marathon runner now living with multiple sclerosis (MS), couldn't participate in his lifelong passion the way he used to.

Yet, by tuning in to his values and passions, he found purpose in advocating for MS research and raising awareness about the illness. His purpose didn't disappear with his diagnosis; it transformed and regenerated in a new form.

## 11.2. Embracing Fulfillment

Fulfillment is inherently personal, an individual journey. It's the deep-seated sense of achievement and happiness stemming from consistently living and nurturing our highest values. It's the contentment that blooms when the gaps between our dreams, values, and realities diminish.

In living with chronic illness, there will be days when physical symptoms are unbearable or when emotional fatigue seeps in. And yet, it's during these moments that the seed of fulfillment can find the most fertile ground to grow. Embrace the challenge of finding joy in the small things, nurturing gratification from aspects of your life that you can control.

Scope out what you can do. If you loved gardening but find it physically demanding now, consider adaptive gardening techniques or indoor plants. If you enjoyed engaging with large groups but find it draining, perhaps smaller, intimate gatherings will suffice. The key is to mold your circumstances to your passions, not the other way around.

## 11.3. The Power of Connection

Chronic illness can be isolating, but purpose and fulfillment often arise from connections. Nurturing relationships with loved ones, forming bonds with people who have similar experiences, or even connecting with professionals in managing your illness, all offer paths to deeper enrichment and meaning.

Linda, living with fibromyalgia, found purpose and fulfillment fostering online communities for individuals with the same condition. Sharing her experiences and creating safe spaces for others to do the same fostered a sense of camaraderie that transcended her personal struggles.

# 11.4. Defying Defeat: Exhibiting Resilience

Living with a chronic illness may shackle you with limitations, but it doesn't mean the end of personal growth. On the contrary, it can provide a wellspring of resilience. Harness this resilience by accepting your circumstances, not as resignations but as acknowledgments of reality. This acceptance is not a sinking into quicksand, it's the ground beneath your feet from which you can leap.

Don't be disheartened if the journey is disorienting at first, it's often the case when charting unfamiliar territory. Be patient with yourself and remember that progress is not linear. Some days may indeed be more challenging than others, but every moment of ardor gives way to learning, growth, and resilience.

# 11.5. Cultivating Mindfulness

Embracing mindfulness merely means actively engaging in the present, acknowledging, and accepting your feelings and experiences without judgment, staying grounded even as the storm of chronic illness swirls around you.

Mindfulness meditation, simple breathing exercises, yoga, or even engaging in a favorite hobby, each provides an avenue to mindfulness. Make a habit of setting aside time for these activities; it's these pockets of peaceful presence that seeds fulfillment and purpose in your life amidst the sea surrounding chronic illness.

# 11.6. The Road Less Traveled

Remember, trials and tribulations are not there to shackle us but to shape us. They are the hammers and chisels sculpting our resilience, the ink with which we write our stories, the dye coloring our tapestries with unique patterns.

Give yourself permission to feel, heal, dream, strive for your goals, and redefine your purpose every day. Chronic illness may have changed the course of your life but remember, you are still its active author, capable, competent, and full of iridescent spirit. After all, it's the road less traveled that makes all the difference. Compassion, connection, resilience, mindfulness, and the pursuit of purpose and fulfillment are your companions on this journey.

Our stories do not end with chronic illness. Rather, they evolve into narrations of courage, endurance, and sheer human spirit. So, go ahead. Write the next chapter. Live passionately. There's a vast scape blooming ahead. The path may be unconventional, but it's undeniably yours.